# Balancing Your Way into Alignment:
## Physical Movement

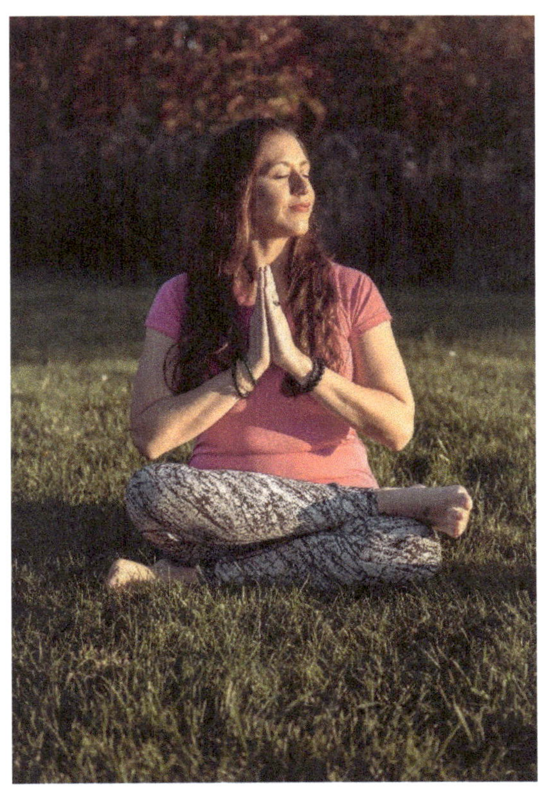

## By Nicole Elko

Photography by Danielle Jean Photography

Image(s) by: Natalie Montgomery



ISBN: 9798866938353

# DEDICATION

To my husband, Tommy, whose encouragement is the wind beneath my wings. Your love, support, and belief in my dreams have been my greatest inspiration. I am filled with gratitude that we are navigating this incredible journey of life side by side. The balance we bring to each other's lives is truly remarkable, and I deeply cherish the shared experiences that have brought us to this moment. While our path may not always be a walk in the park, it's undeniably filled with laughter and adventure.

To my precious children, Asher, Scarlett, and Bodhi, you inspire me every day with your boundless curiosity and joy. Choosing me as your Mother has been a gift beyond measure. It is a role I cherish with all my heart and has fueled my determination to be the best version of myself, setting an example of kindness, resilience, and unconditional love.

To my Mother, Father, Sister, and Brother (Theresa, Michael, Angela, and Victor) your unwavering support, and love is a guiding light through my journey. Each of you has helped shape the person I am today. I am forever grateful for the privilege of having you in my life.

To a mentor and friend, Colleen, your wisdom, guidance, and compassion helped shape my life. Truly words cannot express the immense gratitude I feel for you. Thank you for opening me up to new perspectives, the journey of Self-care and the foundation for loving myself.

To Source, thank you for your guidance to remember my Truth and my own power.

With heartfelt gratitude and love, this book is dedicated to each of you.

# CONTENTS

# ACKNOWLEDGMENTS

To the Oneness: I am filled with immense gratitude for the journey that we embark on together.

# FOREWARD

"Balancing Your Way Into Alignment" is what every human on Earth seeks and Nicole gives us simple, genuine tools to take action. I first met Nicole when she walked into my boutique with gifts and services to promote self-healing. With her love of crystals and desire for balance, Nicole took classes and became the ultimate example for others. Her ability to see the world without judgement and from multiple perspectives makes her an excellent coach for others seeking balance. Many spiritual centers only promote prayer and meditation, but with high frequencies, Indigos, must have movement to regulate and create balance. Knowing this, Nicole volunteered to assist others with movement and meditation classes. Movement is for all people. Although humans often get stuck thinking Yoga is not for them, we know the key to balance is action which means taking care of your physical being, the temple of your soul.

In Nicole's book, "Balancing Your Way into Alignment", Nicole gives us tools for breathing, movement, and use of crystals, to get every person on Earth unstuck, moving, and realizing that Yoga is for everyone. Nicole makes movement easy and allows us to understand the benefit of each pose and crystal while calming our mind, which leads to better health. This outstanding book is for all people seeking wellness and balance. As each person finds love for themselves, peace in families, communities, and the world spread.

Thank you, Nicole, for loving yourself and seeking balance and harmony in yourself and your relationships. You are truly unstoppable and able to get things done. As a seeker of information to improve self and assist others, you know exactly what others need to do to see love in themselves. I love you and am so incredibly proud to call you, my friend. I look forward to sharing this journey with you, spreading peace, harmony, and balance in our community and the world. I encourage all seekers of light and love to get Nicole's book to start their own journey into alignment.

Love,
Colleen Brindley
Author of "Mastering Self"

# Introduction

## TO UNITE, YOKE

Welcome beautiful Soul! I invite you to discover the beautiful world of Yoga, where the mind, body, and soul unite to bring you into a state of peace, balance, and harmony. Rooted in the very essence of its name, yoga, meaning to unite, this ancient practice is all about bringing together the four aspects of Self: the physical, mental, emotional, and spiritual.

Yoga has been around for centuries and has evolved into many different styles, and variations, each with its own unique benefits. From the physical postures known as the asanas to breathing techniques known as pranayama, yoga offers a holistic approach to health and wellness. With numerous benefits, such as increased flexibility, strength, balance, stress relief, and overall wellness, Yoga is embraced by people all over the world.

Yoga is more than physical exercise- it's the journey of self-discovery and self-awareness. Through mindfulness, meditation, and breathwork you will learn how to connect with your body and mind to cultivate inner peace and happiness. Yoga is a practice that has something to offer for everyone. Whether you are looking to improve your physical health, reduce stress and anxiety or deepen your spiritual practice, Yoga can help you achieve your goals.

In the pages that follow, begin an exploration diving into the realm of Yoga and Self. Here, I unveil a tapestry of yoga poses and crystals that will enrich your path toward peace and balance. So, get ready to strike a pose, flip your perspective, and channel your inner balance boss as we explore my handpicked selection of eleven poses that will challenge, empower, and of course, bring a little extra to your practice.

Namafuckingste!

# BREATHWORK

Breathing is one of those things we often take for granted, usually catching ourselves holding our breath. Both in Yoga and throughout life, breathing becomes this incredible tool for both our bodies and minds.

Deep breathing, a key technique, involves slow, deliberate inhalations that fill your lungs with oxygen. It's like a mini life boost! It doesn't just help your blood flow better; it's like a stressbuster, too. Super helpful in everyday life.

What's fascinating is how deep breathing activates our relaxation system. Its ability to lower stress levels and anxiety is truly remarkable. Additionally, it serves as a workout for the lungs and actively engages the heart. However, the true marvel lies in its versatility – it's not merely about relaxation. Deep breathing can also be harnessed to manage pain, enhance sleep quality, and provide a genuine surge of energy.

If you want to give it a shot, find a comfy spot, sit up straight (no slouching!), and close your eyes. It's like a mini relaxation ritual, and it's awesome once you get the hang of it! If you want to take your breathing up a notch, there are a couple of cool tricks to try. First up, there's diaphragmatic breathing. Your diaphragm is the muscle right below your lungs that's the boss of your breathing. So, when you take a deep breath in, let your belly puff out like a balloon, filling your lungs from the bottom up. Then, as you breathe out, feel your belly flatten as you push the air out from the bottom, kind of like deflating a balloon. Another technique, timing. Try inhaling for a flow count of four, hold that breath for two, and then exhale nice and east for a count of six. It's like a little magic trick that can calm your nervous system and zap away stress. The last technique, pursed lip breathing. Inhale slowly through your nose for a count of two. Exhale through pursed lips as if you were blowing out a candle for four counts. Give these a try, and you'll feel peaceful and calm in no time.

# FOUR ASPECTS OF SELF

Yoga is essentially connected to the four-fold being, the physical, spiritual, mental, and emotional aspects of our existence. This ancient practice is a holistic journey that unites these dimensions, allowing us to explore and harmonize every facet of our being. Experimenting with Yoga marked the beginning of my journey towards self-discovery and well-being. Here, I recognized the intricate interconnectedness of our existence and the significance of cultivating a self-care routine. By nurturing these aspects of Self harmoniously, leads to a more fulfilled and balanced life.

## Fostering Physical Vitality

Our physical well-being is the vessel that carries us through life's journey. By prioritizing regular exercise, our body and mind become strong and energized. Maintaining a balanced diet rich in nutrients, hydration, and mindful eating habits while getting enough sleep rejuvenates our body and mind to assist with better focus. Stepping onto the Yoga mat is an adventure. Each pose, a puzzle piece, as you try them out you learn about your body's unique capabilities, strengths, and areas that need nurturing. Here, you discover your inner flexibility and further develop the strength that resides within. Small habits lead to significant improvements in your physical health over time.

## Nourishing Mental Clarity

A well-nurtured mind is key to unlocking your full potential. By engaging in lifelong learning helps keep your mental faculties sharp. Practice mindfulness to stay present and manage stress. Practicing mindfulness involves being fully present in the moment, observing your thoughts and sensations without judgement. Instead of getting caught up in your thoughts, simply observe them as if they were clouds passing through the sky. While on the mat, you grant yourself the chance to exist entirely in the present moment. If you observe your mind drifting, perhaps on your action list or a specific situation, no worries! Offer yourself compassion and gently return your focus to your breath. Embrace creativity through hobbies and activities that stimulate your imagination.

## Encompassing Emotional Wholeness

Our emotions are the vibrant colors that paint the canvas of our lives. To care for our emotional well-being, practice self-awareness, emotional intelligence, and self-compassion. Allow yourself to feel and express your emotions, whether high vibrational or low vibrational, while learning healthy ways to cope with your emotions. Cultivate healthy relationships that provide support, empathy, and understanding. Surround yourself with positive influences and seek a community of friends and family that you vibe with. Strive for balance in your life. Acknowledge that your emotions are an integral part of who you are and find ways to live authentically. A well-rounded lifestyle that includes physical health, mental well-being, and social connections contributes to emotional wellness.

## Tending to Spiritual Wellness

Our spiritual well-being forms the foundation of your four-fold being. It's about connecting with our inner self and the universe around us. Engage in practices that resonate with you, such as meditation, prayers, or spending time in nature. Reflect on your values, purpose, and the meaning you find in life. Nurture a sense of gratitude and strive for inner peace and mindfulness.

## The Integration of Self

True well-being emerges when we harmonize these dimensions. Combining the physical, spiritual, mental, and emotional aspects of our being leads to a profound sense of balance and purpose. As you set out on this journey, remember that it is a dynamic process. Regular self-assessment and adjustments are crucial are you navigate life's ever-changing landscape. Remember, each dimension is interconnected, and neglecting one aspect may affect the others. By paying attention to and caring for all four aspects of your being, you create a harmonious and balanced life.

## Encouraging Consistency

Caring for your four-fold being is an ongoing commitment. Set goals for each aspect of your being and develop consistency in your practice. Ensure that you allocate time and energy to each dimension. Create a holistic daily routine that includes moments of self-reflection, self-expression, and physical activity.

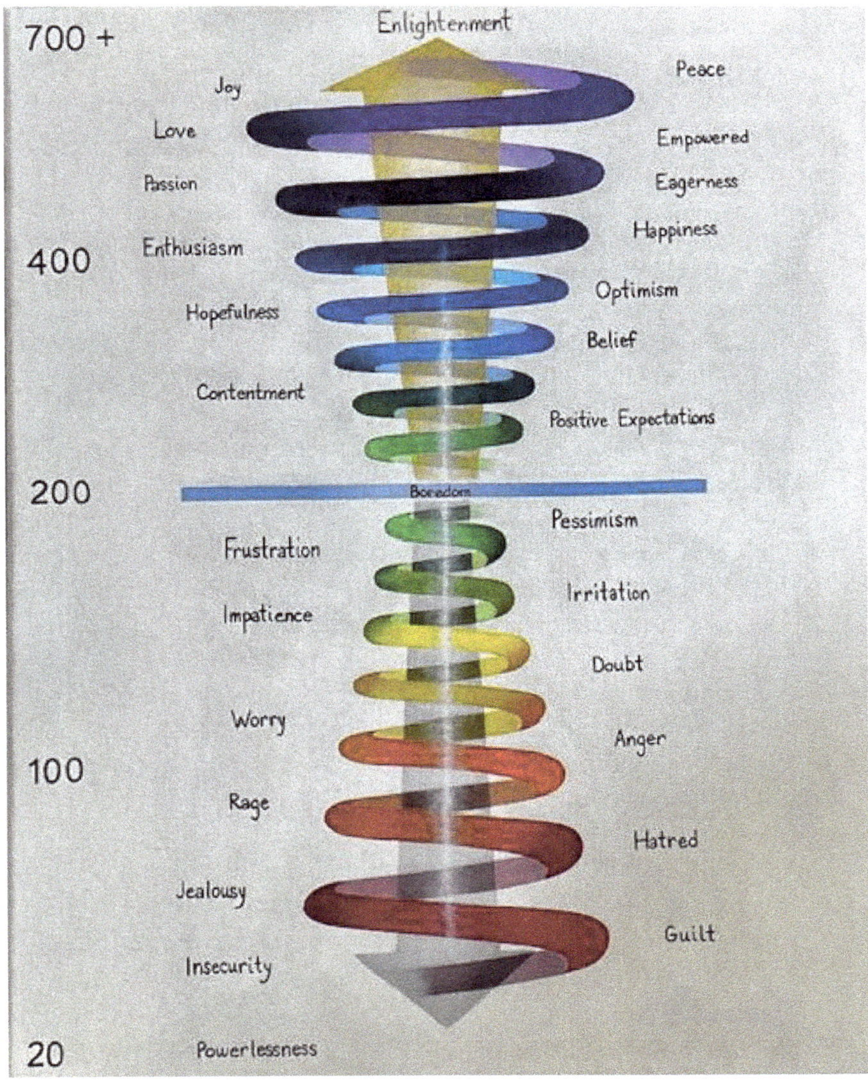

# ZEN-IFYING YOUR ZONE

To really get the most out of your Yoga practice, it's super important to clear your mind and find your center. When you do this, it's like waving goodbye to all the day's stress and saying hello to a deep connection with your body, breath, and mind. Now, finding your center means zeroing in on your core, right around your belly, which is also known as the solar plexus chakra. This is where your energy and strength hang out. When you connect with this spot, you tap into your inner power and wisdom, making it easier to move and breathe gracefully. You'll also feel more grounded, calm, and peaceful. Centering yourself helps you stay in the moment and connect with your true self. The result? More harmony and balance in the body, mind, and spirit.

Before you dive into your practice, here are some easy tips to clear your head and center yourself:

Find Your Zone: Seek out a quiet, interruption-free space. Silence your phone and ditch the TV. Make it comfy and cozy.

Chill and Breathe: Get comfy on the floor. Take some deep breaths, in through your nose, out through your mouth. Focus on your breath and let go of any random thoughts or worries.

Set an Intention: Before you start, set an intention for your practice. It could be anything that vibes with you, like peace, strength, or gratitude. Take a moment to think about it and keep it in mind throughout your practice.

Mindfulness Magic: Practice mindfulness, which means being in the moment and watching your thoughts and feelings without judging. Pay attention to your breath and the present moment. If your mind drifts away, gently steer it back to your breath.

Aromatherapy Bonus: Essential oils or incense can help create a calming atmosphere. Scents like lavender, frankincense, sandalwood, and Release oils are awesome for Yoga. Use a diffuser or light some incense before you start to set the mood.

Taking a few moments to clear your head and center yourself will make your practice feel more grounded, focused, and present. Just be patient and always listen to your body.

"The exceptional person you see in the mirror is you!" – Source

# "All of you can change yourself and your Earth. WE believe in You."- Source

# CHAPTER 1

# HULA HOOP POSE

## POSE BENEFITS:
Stretches the glutes, hamstrings, quadriceps, pelvic floor muscles, lower back, and abdominal muscles.

## CRYSTAL:
Citrine- cleanses aura, activates creativity, promotes a sense of security, and helps to see the bright side of things.

## CHAKRA:
Sacral

# Hula Hoop Pose

1. Stand in the middle of your mat with your feet hip-width apart and your hand in prayer position or on your hips.
2. Ground through your feet spreading your toes and engaging your core.
3. Move your hips in a circular motion towards the right for 7 deep full breaths by inhaling slowly for a count of 3 and exhaling slowly for a count of 3.
4. Come back to the center.
5. Move your hips in a circular motion towards the left for 7 deep full breaths by inhaling slowly for a count of 3 and exhaling slowly for a count of 3.

## CRYSTAL:

Citrine- cleanses aura, activates creativity, promotes a sense of security, and helps to see the bright side of things.

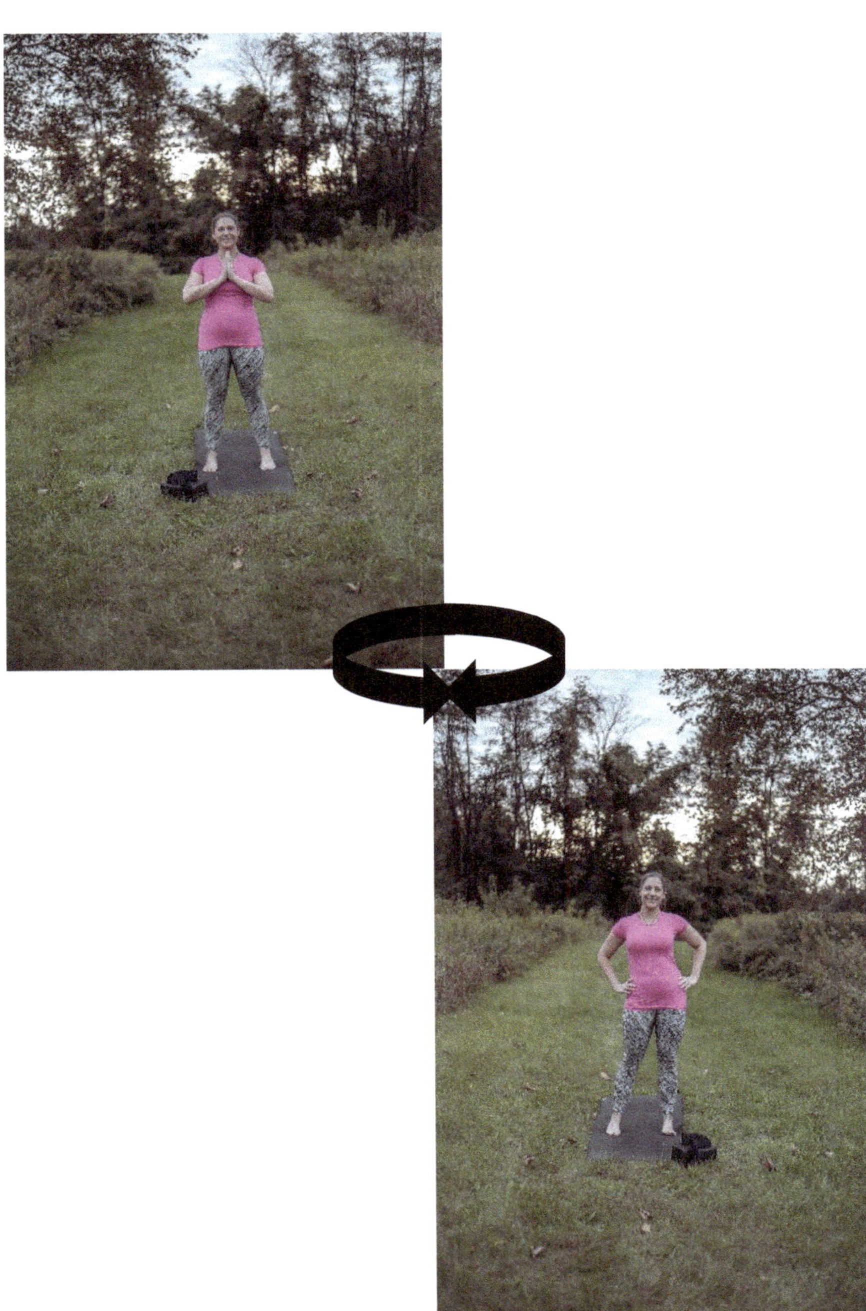

# "Your smile has power, great power." - Source

# CHAPTER 2

# DIAMOND REACH POSE

## POSE BENEFITS:
Stretches strengthen, and lengthens groin, inner thighs, and knees. Strengthens pelvic floor muscles, psoas, and hip flexors allowing for a greater range of flexibility and motion.

## CRYSTAL:
Aquamarine- Calms nerves, reduces, and relieves stress.

## CHAKRA:
Throat

# Diamond Reach Pose

1. Sit on the mat with knees bent, feet flat hip-width distance apart.
2. Place hands by hips, fingers pointing towards feet.
3. Lift feet, keeping knees bent, and bringing soles of your feet together.
4. Thread hands between knees.
5. Inhale slowly for a count of 3 and exhale slowly for a count of 3.
6. Repeat 7 times.
7. To release the pose, lower your legs and release hands.

## CRYSTAL:

Aquamarine- Calms nerves, reduces, and relieves stress.

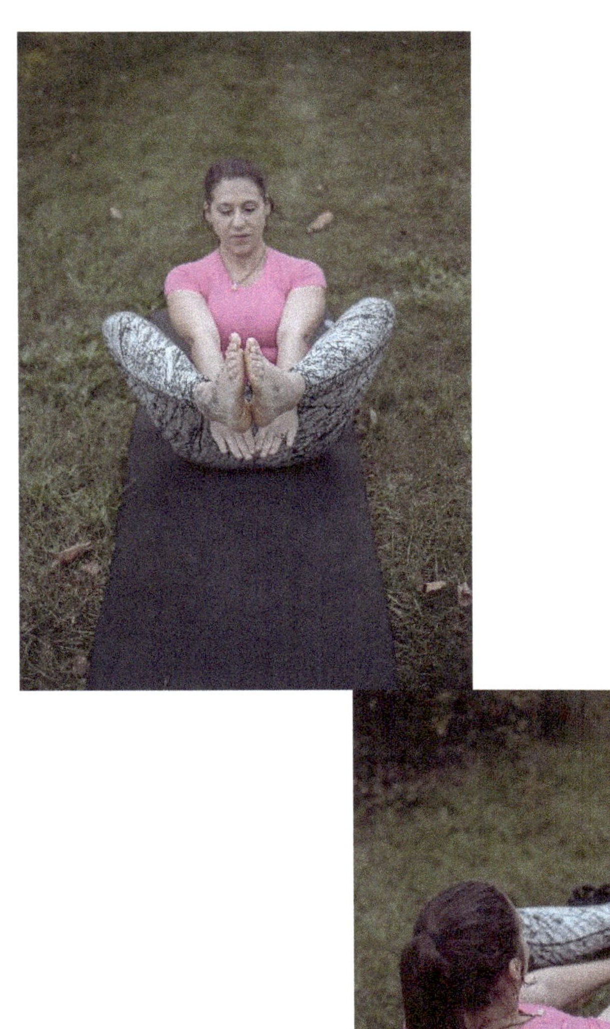

# Diamond Reach Pose- Variation

1. Sit on the mat, gently bend your knees and press the soles of your feet together.
2. Stretch your arms towards the edge of your mat.
3. Inhale slowly for a count of 3 and exhale slowly for a count of 3.
4. Repeat 7 times.

## CRYSTAL:

Aquamarine- Calms nerves, reduces, and relieves stress.

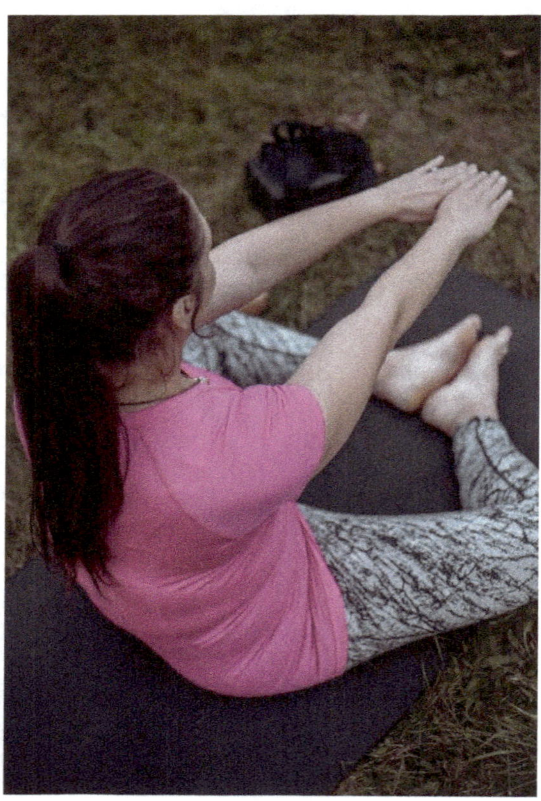

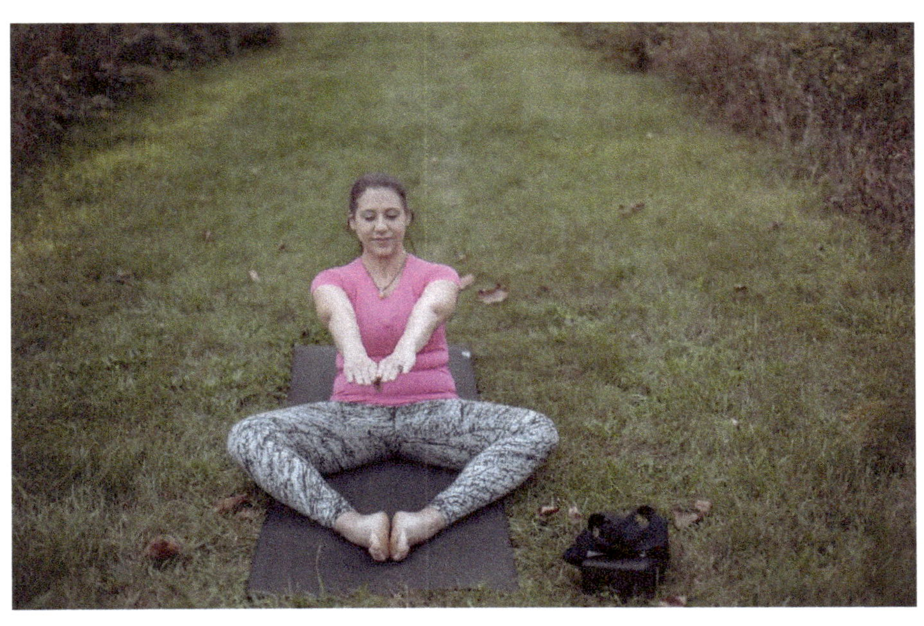

"All of you desire to be liked by your others; and well you should. However, you don't need anyone's approval, and they don't need yours. This is a fact! Accept it and your vibration will change. You will draw towards you those of Like Mind." – Source

# CHAPTER 3

# BUTTERFLY TWIST POSE

## POSE BENEFITS:
Strengthens the pelvic floor, psoas muscles, and hip flexors.

## CRYSTAL:
Calcite – mental and emotional balance, emotional release, and calming.

## CHAKRA:
Throat and Third Eye

# Butterfly Twist Pose

1. Sit on the mat with legs extended.
2. Bend knees, and place soles of feet together
3. Sit tall and lengthen spine. *Imagine a string being pulled up through the crown of your head.*
4. Exhale twist left, right arm across knee and left arm towards the sky. Gently inhale for a count of 3 and exhale for a count of 3. To deepen the pose, stay here for 7 breaths.
5. Slowly inhale and come back through the center.
6. Exhale twist right, left arm across knee and right arms towards the sky. Gently inhale for a count of 3 and exhale for a count of 3. To deepen the pose, stay here for 7 breaths.

## CRYSTAL:

Calcite – mental and emotional balance, emotional release, and calming.

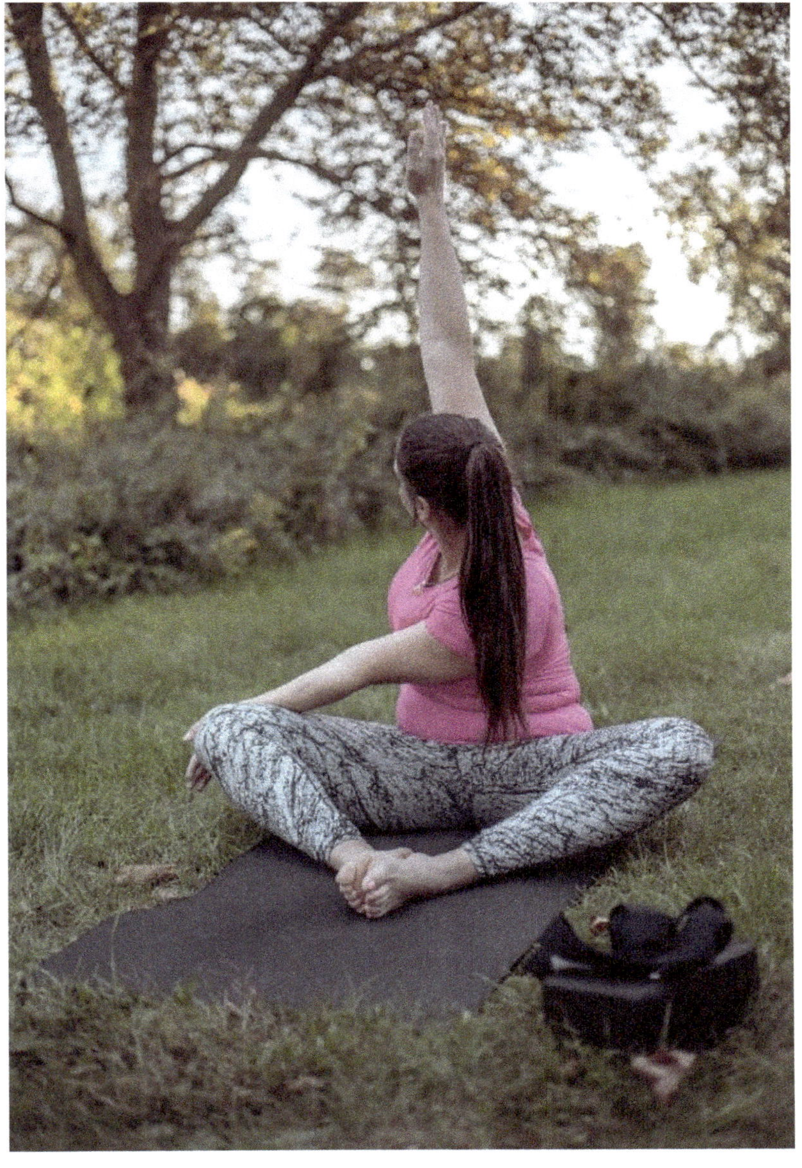

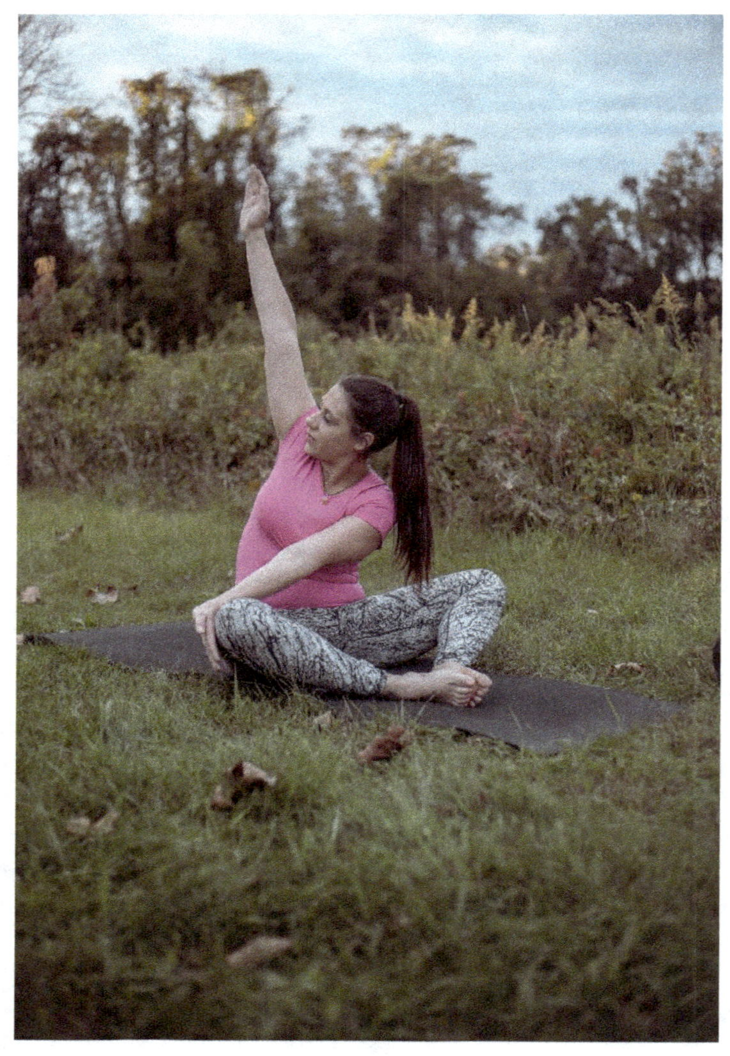

25

**"Open your mind to the truth of the matter- You Matter, you belong, and you are as magnificent as the stars above."**

**– Source**

CHAPTER 4

# ENERGIZING RELEASE POSE

## POSE BENEFITS:
Increases energy throughout the body, stretches the arms, shoulders, core, biceps, and triceps.

## CRYSTAL:
Unakite- converts negativity, promotes positive vibes, ignites compassion and peace within.

## CHAKRA:
Heart

# Energizing Release Pose

## Breathwork: (Optional)

1. To begin the pose, exhale forcefully and rapidly through your nose, activating your diaphragm to push the air out. The inhalation will naturally ensue as the diaphragm returns to a relaxed state.
2. Maintain a steady and unbroken rhythm for your breaths. Both inhalation and exhalation should last for an equal duration, with the focus on the vigorous exhale.
3. While exhaling, your belly will naturally contract inward, and during inhalation, it will naturally expand outward.

## This is a dynamic movement.

1. Stand on your mat with your feet slightly wider than the width of your hips. Slowly inhale through your nose and raise your arms above your head.
2. Exhale with force, like you're blowing out a candle, at the same time energetically sweep your arms down past your sides and bend at your knees to sit back into your hips (squat stance).
3. Slowly inhale through your nose. Push through your heels and extend your legs to stand up straight and raise your arms toward the sky. Repeat 7 times.

## CRYSTAL:

Unakite- converts negativity, promotes positive vibes, ignites compassion and peace within.

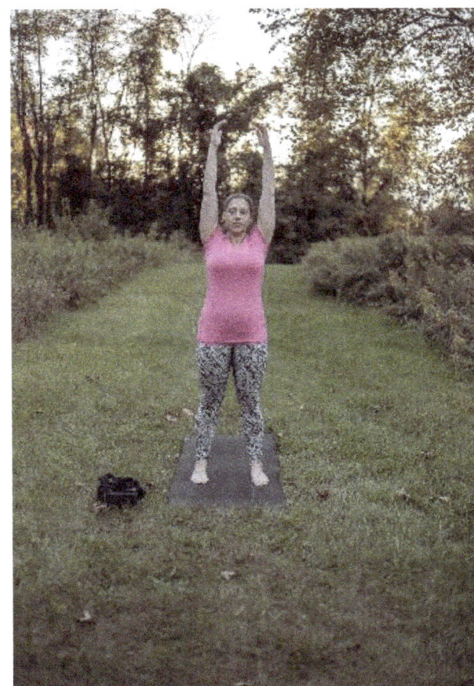

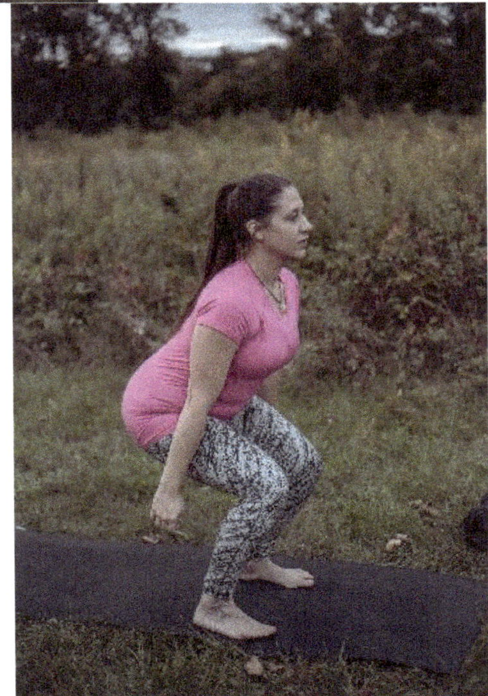

"You are capable of great things within and outside of your physical being."

– Source

# CHAPTER 5

# WINDSHIELD WIPER OPENING POSE

## POSE BENEFITS:
Stretches IT band, quadriceps, glutes, abdominal muscles, psoas, and lower back.

## CRYSTAL:
Howlite- discernment, ability to perceive and understand.

## CHAKRA:
Crown

# Windshield Wiper Opening Pose

1. Sit on the mat with your knees slightly bent hip-width distance apart, soles of your feet on the floor.
2. Bring your arms behind you, palms flat on the mat, fingers pointed toward the front of the mat.
3. Gently exhale your knees to the right.
4. Sit up tall and lengthen spine. *Imagine a string being pulled up through the crown of your head.*
5. As you begin to inhale, clasp your hands behind your back and slide your hands towards your left hip.
6. Remain here for 7 breaths.
7. Repeat on opposite side.

## CRYSTAL:

Howlite- discernment, ability to perceive and understand.

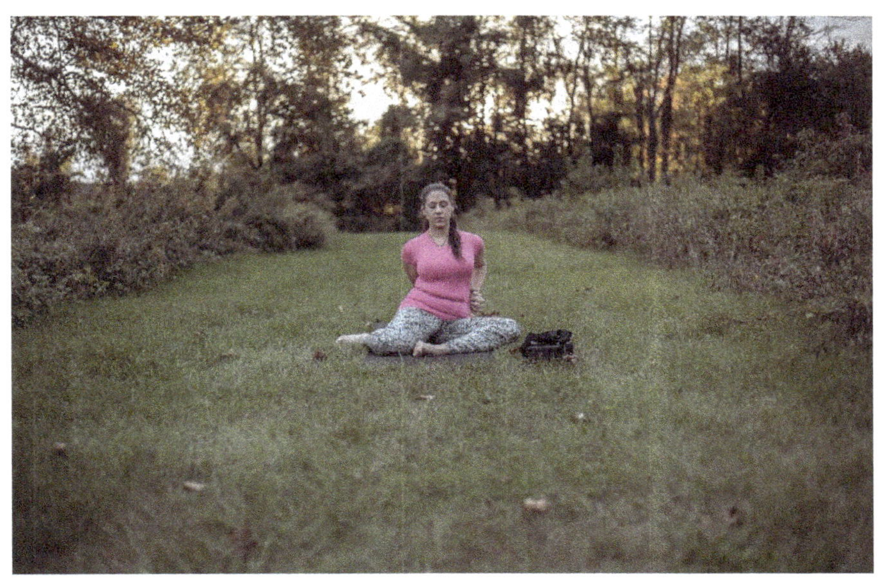

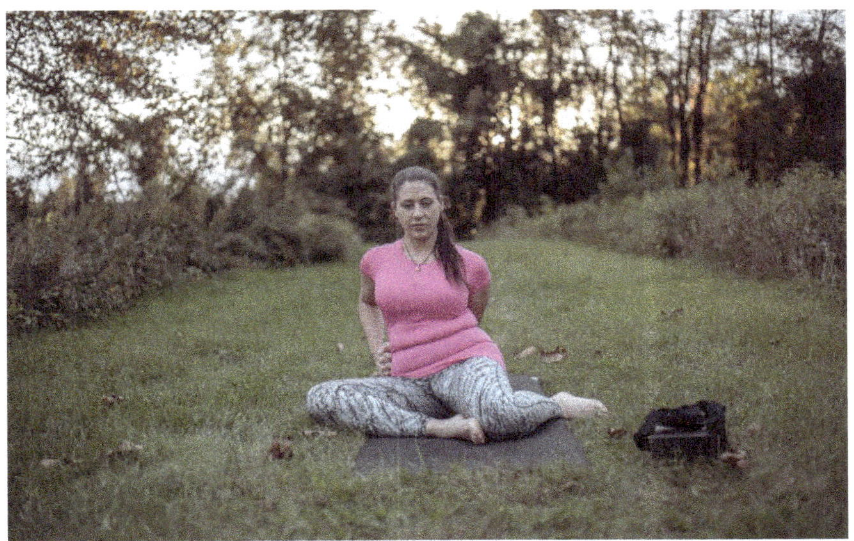

"I AM self-sustaining. I AM able
to take care of Self. This includes
my body, mind, and spirit."
- Source

CHAPTER 6

# STANDING HARMONY POSE

## POSE BENEFITS:
Stretches hip muscles, hamstrings, and quadriceps.
Strengthens the grounding leg.

## CRYSTAL:
Peridot- personal growth, transformation, and encouraging
a positive outlook.

## CHAKRA:
Solar Plexus

# Standing Harmony Pose

1. Stand with feet hip-width distance apart.
2. Shift your weight to your left foot.
3. Raise your right knee towards the sky.
4. Slide your right arm beneath your knee and hold onto your ankle.
5. Lift left arm straight out towards the side.
6. Gently inhale for a count of 3 and exhale for a count of 3. To deepen the pose, stay here for 7 breaths.
7. Repeat on opposite side.

## CRYSTAL:

Peridot- personal growth, transformation, and encouraging a positive outlook.

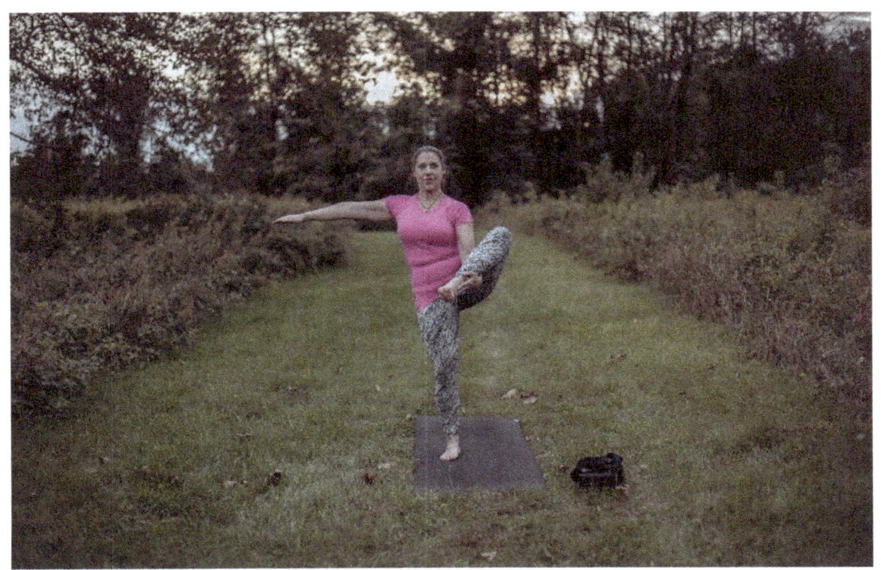

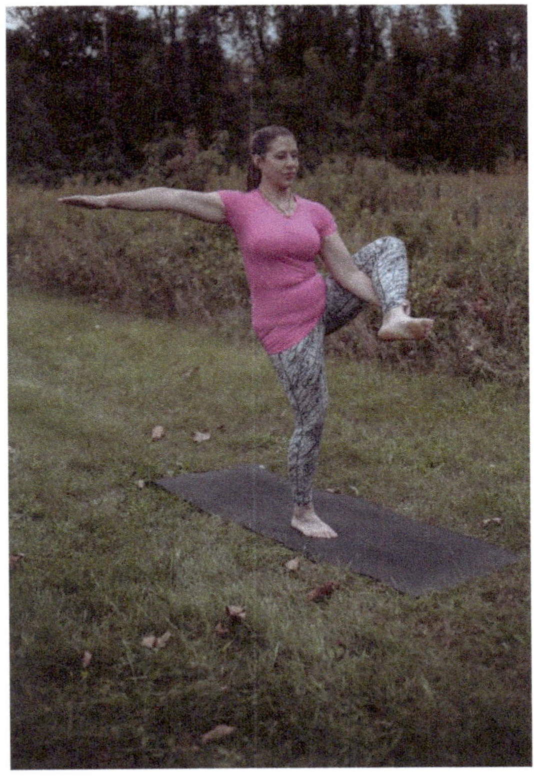

# "I AM Light.
# I AM Love" - Source

# CHAPTER 7

# FORWARD ARM STRETCH POSE

## POSE BENEFITS:
Stretches hamstrings, calves, lower back, arms, and shoulders.

## CRYSTAL:
Onyx- relieves stress.

## CHAKRA:
Root

# Forward Arm Stretch Pose

1. Begin in a standing position, feet together and arms at your side.
2. Slowly inhale through the nose, interlace your fingers behind your back and lift your heart towards the sky expanding your chest.
3. Slowly exhale through the mouth, hinge at the hips and fold forward.
4. Gently inhale for a count of 3 and exhale for a count of 3. Stay here for 7 breaths.
5. Release the arms, slowly roll up one vertebra at a time.

## CRYSTAL:
Onyx- relieves stress.

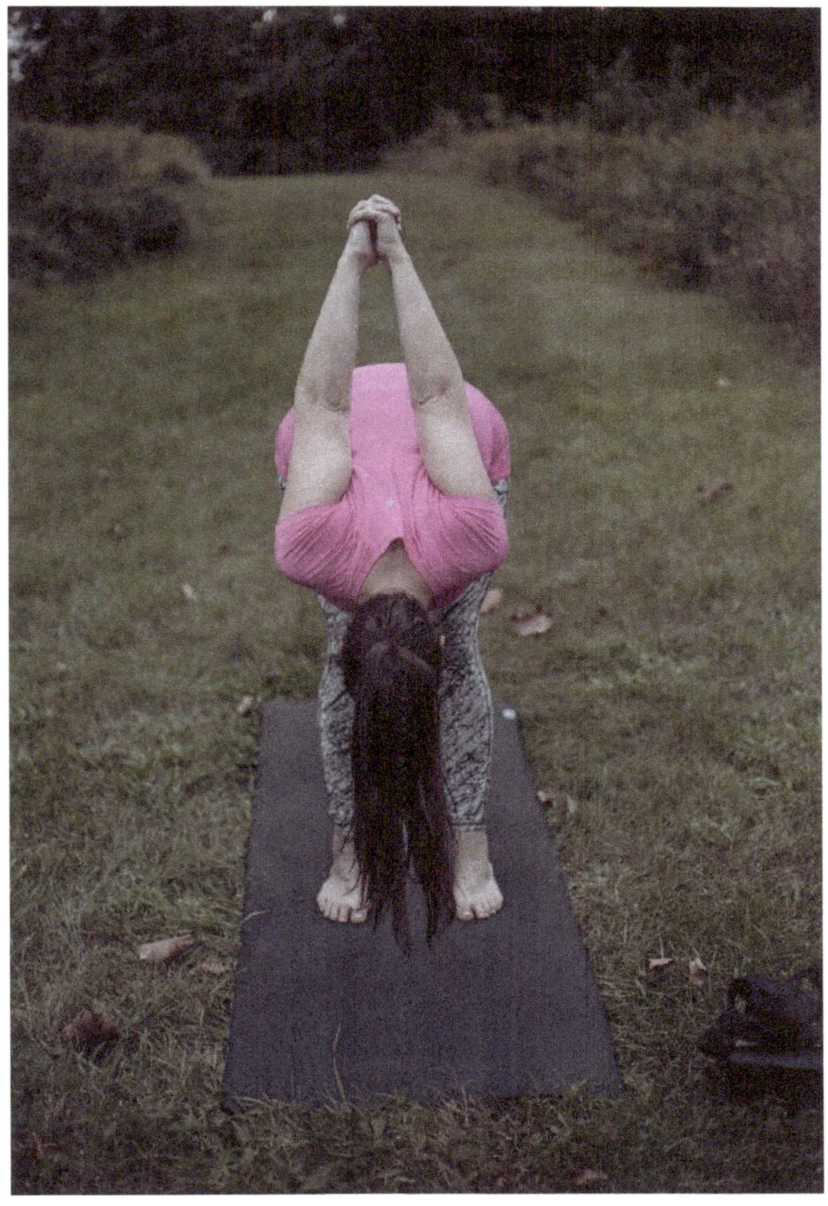

# Forward Arm Stretch Pose Variation

1. Begin in a standing position, feet together and arms at your side.
2. Slowly inhale through the nose, hinge at the hips.  Slowly exhale through the mouth and fold forward.
3. Lift your arms behind you towards the sky.
4. Gently inhale for a count of 3 and exhale for a count of 3. Stay here for 7 breaths.
5. Release the arms, slowly roll up one vertebra at a time.

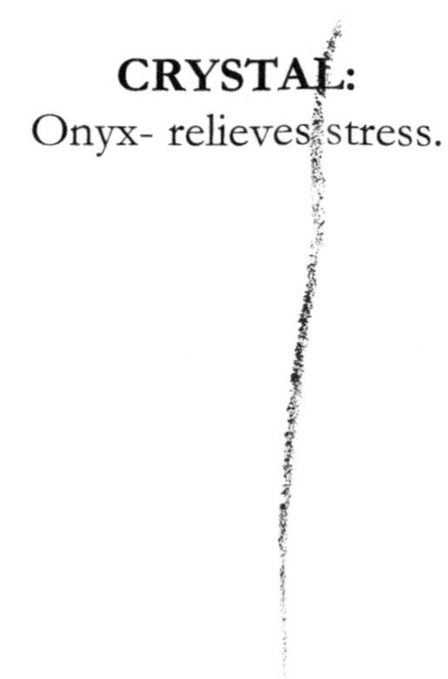

## CRYSTAL:
Onyx- relieves stress.

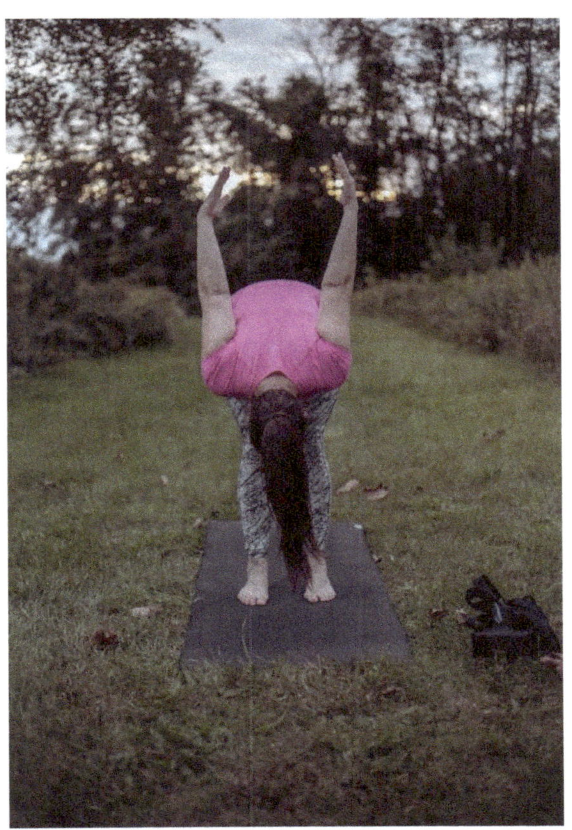

"Remember, it is the rain that causes flowers to grow. It is you that brings smiles to the faces of the ones that you love." - Source

# CHAPTER 8

# FLYING TREE POSE

## POSE BENEFITS:
Combination of balance, stability, strength, stretch, and focus. Stretches and strengthens the leg muscles, hips, core, arms, back muscles, and shoulder muscles.

## CRYSTAL:
Garnet- balances energy flow.

## CHAKRA:
Root and Heart

# Flying Tree Pose

## This is a dynamic pose.
1. Begin in a standing position hip-width distance apart.
2. Shift your weight onto the right foot.
3. Lift the left leg off the ground placing the sole of the foot on the inner thigh, (variation: place sole of foot on calf or ankle) of your standing leg. **Do not place your foot on your knee.**
4. Find your balance by selecting a focal point on the floor and tighten your core.
5. Bring your hands into prayer position at your chest.
6. Breathe and on an exhale extend your arms to the side and your left foot out in front of you.
7. Slowly inhale, bring your hands back into prayer position and the sole of your foot onto your inner thigh, calf, or ankle.
8. Repeat this sequence 7 times.
9. Repeat on opposite sides.

## CRYSTAL:
Garnet- Balances energy flow.

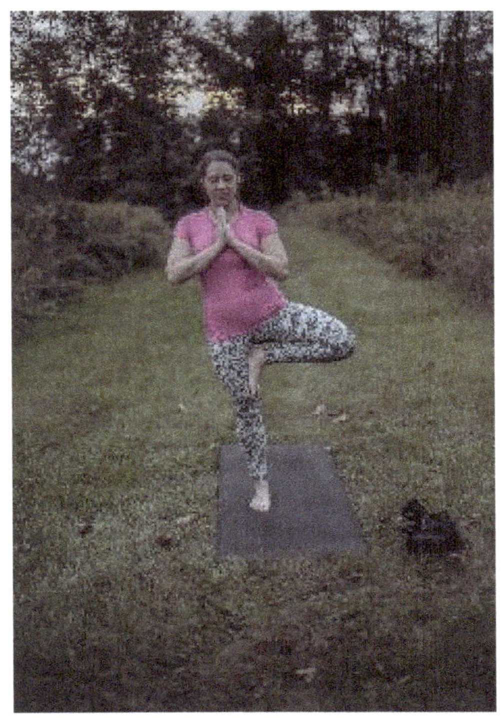

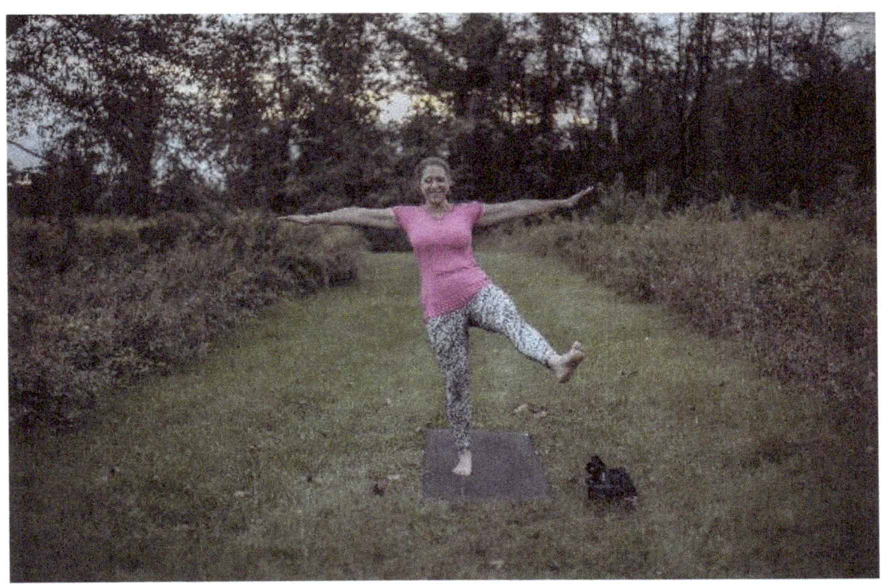

# Flying Tree Pose - Variations

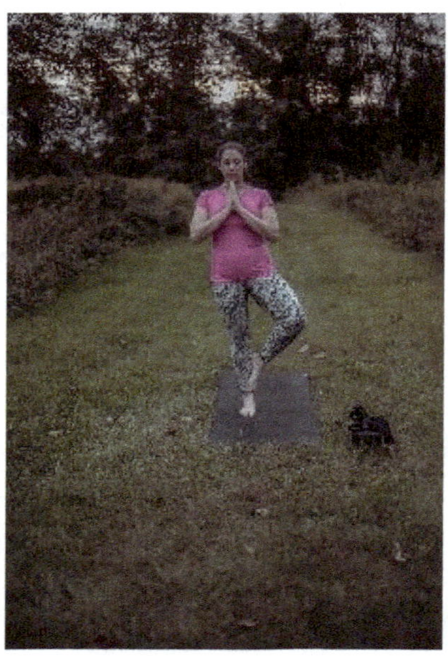

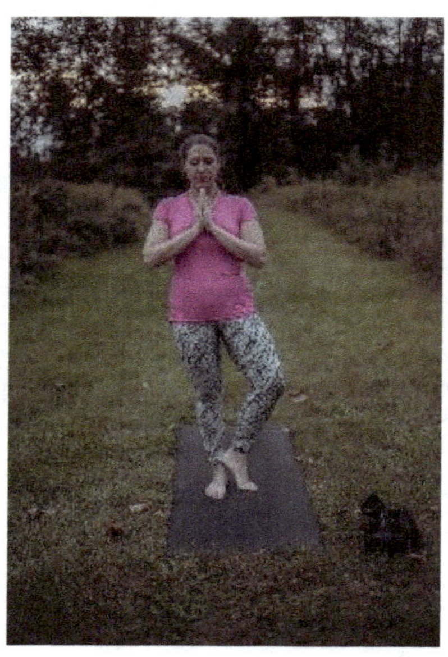

"Even when it seems dark there is always **LIGHT**. Even when you feel there is no hope there is **LOVE**." – Source

CHAPTER 9

# TWISTED ONE KNEE UP POSE

## POSE BENEFITS:

Strengthens ankle, knee, hip joints, calves, and hamstrings.
Stretches glutes, hamstrings, calves, and quadriceps.

## CRYSTAL:

Angelite- strengthening.

## CHAKRA:

Solar Plexus

# Twisted One Knee Up Pose

1. Stand on your mat, feet hip-width distance apart, arms at your side.
2. Slowly inhale, raise your right knee towards the sky.
3. Slowly exhale, rotate your torso towards the right, open your arms in opposite directions looking over your right shoulder.
4. Gently inhale for a count of 3 and exhale for a count of 3. Stay here for 7 breaths.
5. Repeat on opposite side.

**CRYSTAL:**

Angelite- strengthening.

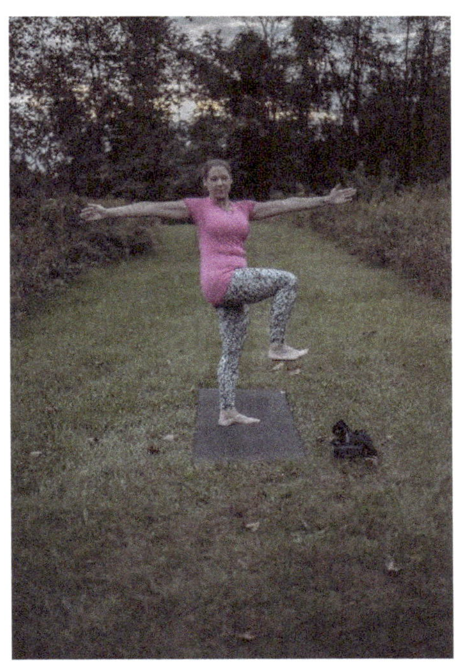

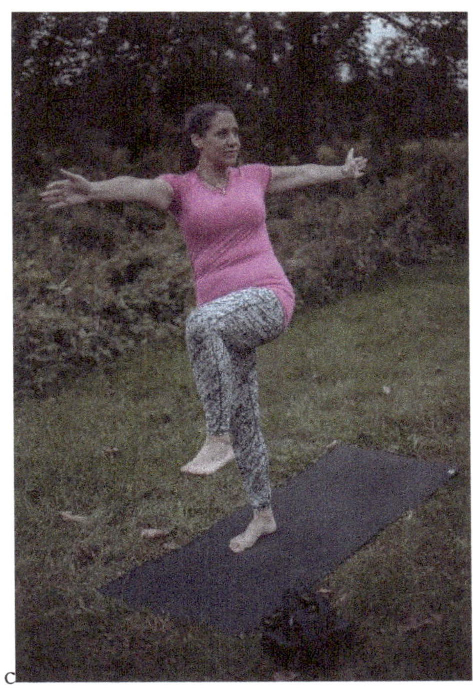

"It is at those times when you think you have no answers and you think you do not know which way to go that if you but try, the creator in you will step forth and give you the faith to carry yourself on into another day." - Source

CHAPTER 10

# EMBRACE POSE

**POSE BENEFITS:**
Enhances the flexibility of the hamstrings, thighs, and hip flexors. Tones, strengthens, and balances energy.

**CRYSTAL:**
Amethyst- promotes positivity.

**CHAKRA:**
Heart

# Embrace Pose

1. Sit with legs extended.
2. Slowly inhale through the nose, adjust your seat to make sure you are on your sit bones.
3. Slowly exhale through the mouth and fold forward.
4. Wrap your arms under your knees and hold opposite elbows. (Variation: If you cannot hold opposite elbows, clasp your hands.)
5. Bend your head towards your thighs.
6. Gently inhale for a count of 3 and exhale for a count of 3. Stay here for 7 breaths.

## CRYSTAL:

Amethyst- promotes positivity.

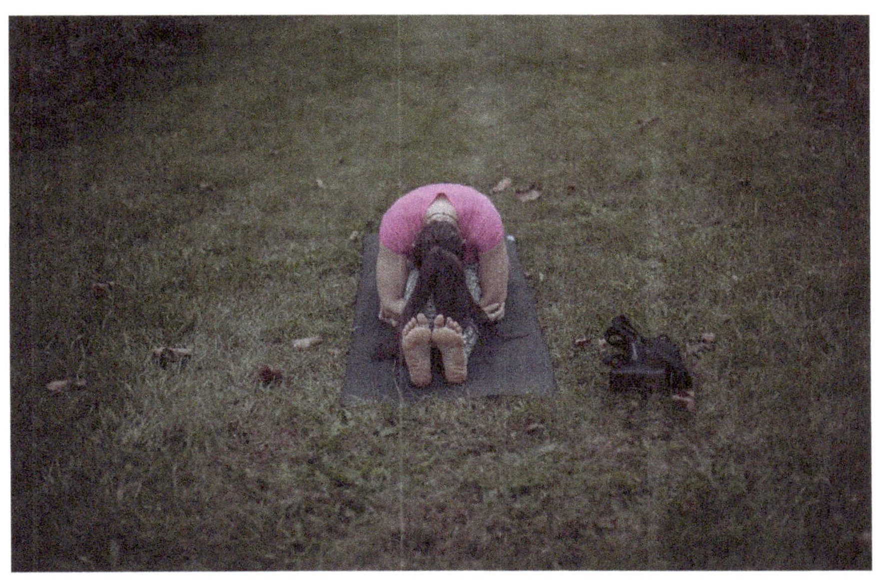

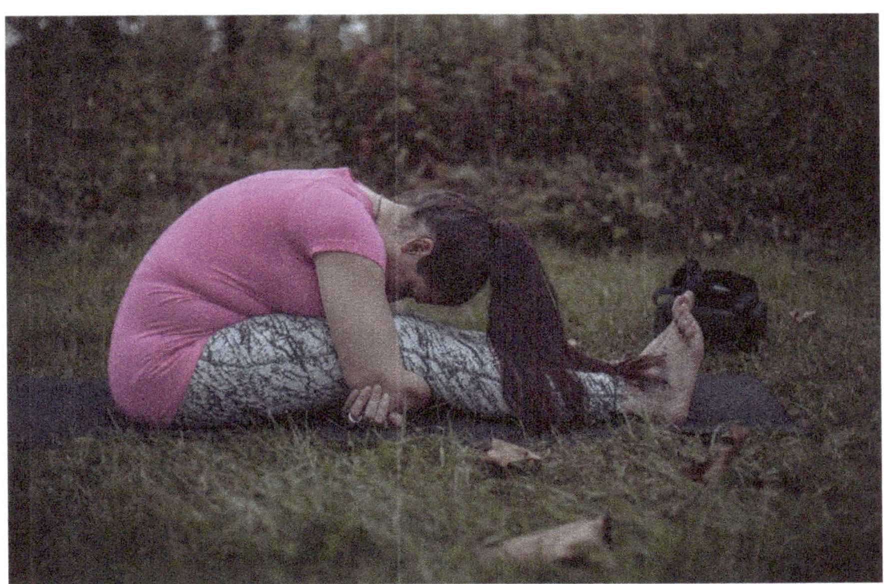

# "You need to understand that you are Perfect, just as you are." - Source

CHAPTER 11

# STANDING TALL POSE

## POSE BENEFITS:
Promotes calmness and mindfulness. Improves flexibility and balance. Stretches hip flexors, calves, quadriceps, triceps, and biceps.

## CRYSTAL:
Kyanite- clarity

## CHAKRA:
Crown

# Standing Tall Pose

1. Stand on your mat, feet hip-width distance apart, arms at your side.
2. Slowly inhale, raise your right knee towards the sky.
3. Slowly exhale, grab the outside of your right foot with your right hand.
4. Find your balance by selecting a focal point on the floor and lift your left arm towards the sky.
5. Gently inhale for a count of 3 and exhale for a count of 3. Stay here for 7 breaths.
6. Repeat on opposite side.

**CRYSTAL:**

Kyanite- clarity

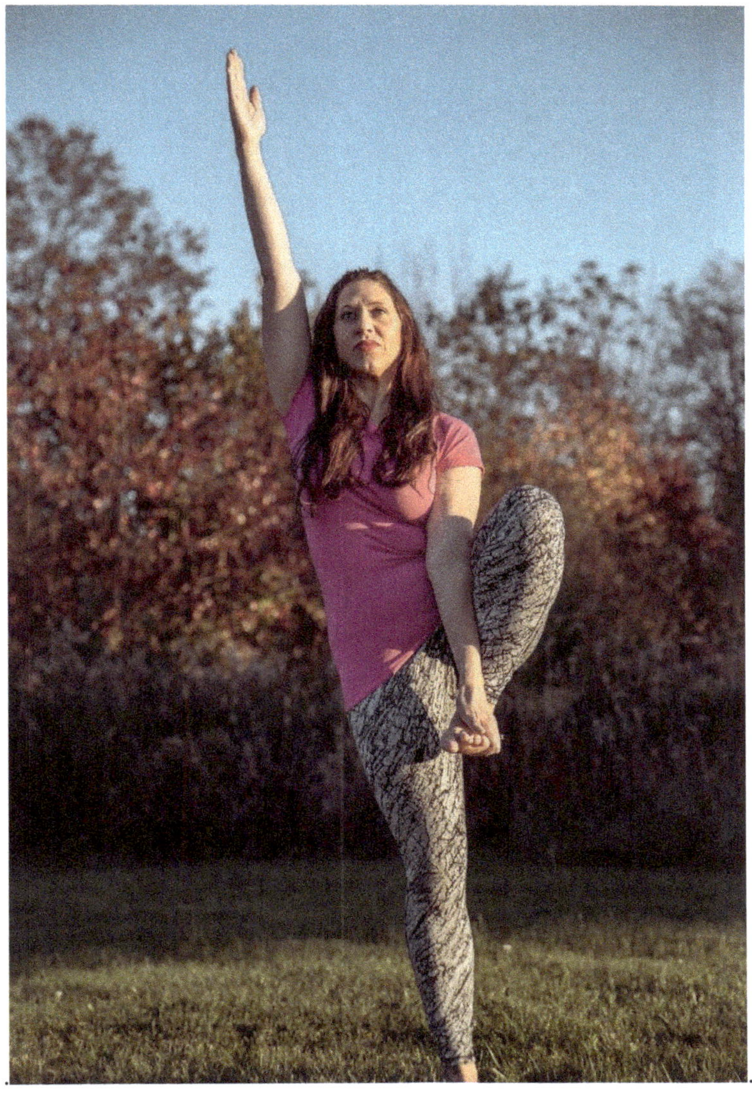

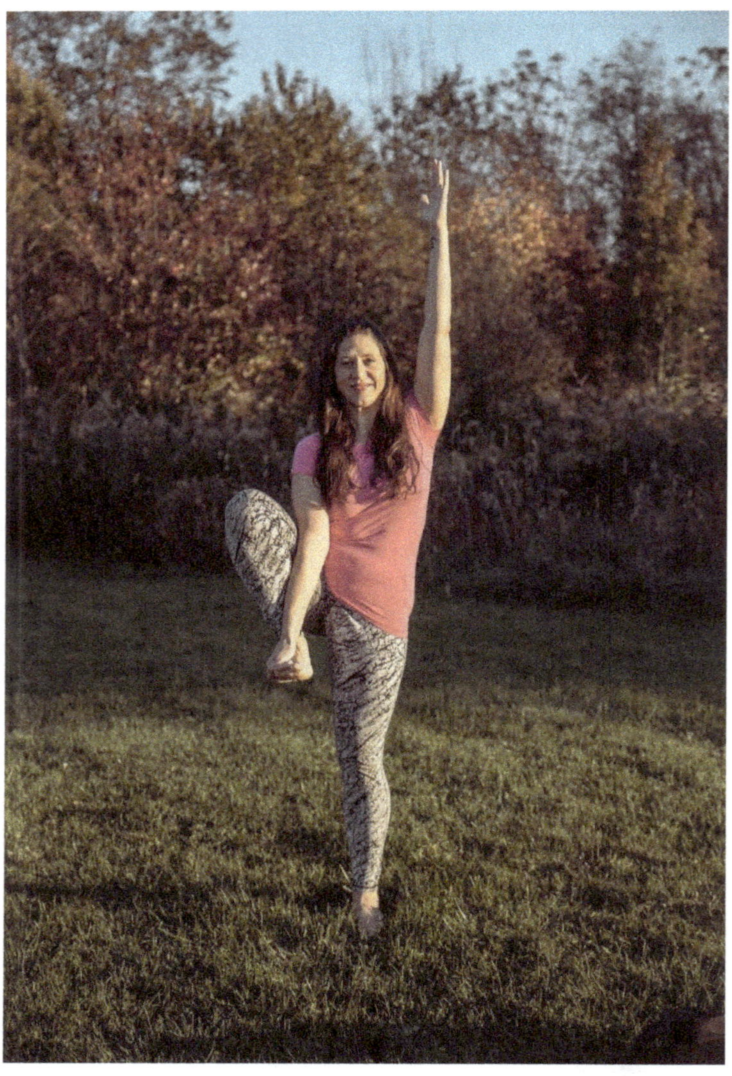

"It is imperative to note that the concept of Negativity is not natural. Unhappiness is not in your makeup. It has been created by the human mental and reinforced by the emotional. Just like the song, "Don't worry, Be Happy!"- Source

# FINAL THOUGHTS

As we conclude this journey through the pages of "Balancing Your Way into Alignment", I invite you to reflect on the life-changing power of Yoga, the art of caring for your four-fold being, and the commitment to balancing Self. In this book, we explored eleven poses that allow us to achieve balance in our lives. Balance is about being open and honest with ourselves to recognize the areas in our lives that require our attention and focus.

Balance is all about tuning into every part of who you are. And the thing is, it's not a one-size fits all deal. It will change from person to person, and even for you as you go through different phases of life. And that's absolutely okay! We are not here to compete with anyone else's journey; it's about embracing our own path, living in the present, and savoring every moment.

Our job, if you ask me, is to be the best version of ourselves, not just for our own sake but to be a shining light in this world. Because when we change and grow, we ripple those positive changes out into the world.

By taking care of our physical selves, we're not just raising our own vibes, but we are also lifting up others around us.

May you continue to walk the path of self-discovery, health, and well-being, finding balance in every moment. It's like this beautiful, interconnected dance where we are all in it together, helping each other shine a bit brighter.

**With much love and gratitude!**

**Nicole Elko**